Acid Reflux

How To Treat Acid Reflux
How To Prevent Acid Reflux

By Ace McCloud
Copyright © 2014

Disclaimer

The information provided in this book is designed to provide helpful information on the subjects discussed. This book is not meant to be used, nor should it be used, to diagnose or treat any medical condition. For diagnosis or treatment of any medical problem, consult your own physician. The publisher and author are not responsible for any specific health or allergy needs that may require medical supervision and are not liable for any damages or negative consequences from any treatment, action, application or preparation, to any person reading or following the information in this book. Any references included are provided for informational purposes only. Readers should be aware that any websites or links listed in this book may change.

Table of Contents

Introduction 6

Chapter 1: Acid Reflux Disease: What Fuels the Fire? 7

Chapter 2: How to Prevent Acid Reflux Disease 9

Chapter 3: Medical Solutions: When Enough is Enough ... 14

Chapter 4: All Natural and Alternative Solutions 19

Chapter 5: Exercise: The Skinny on the Burn 25

Chapter 6: Dietary Solutions 27

Chapter 7: Water: Tap In or Tap Out 29

Conclusion 31

My Other Books and Audio Books 32

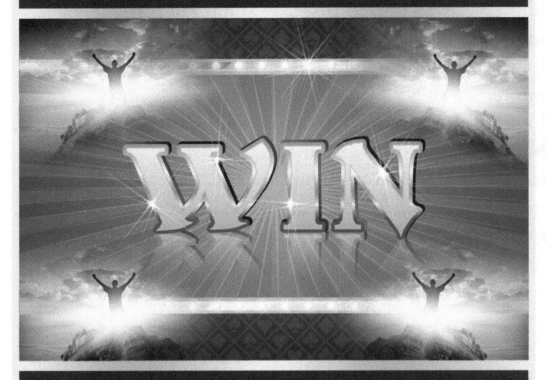

DEDICATED TO THOSE WHO ARE PLAYING THE GAME OF LIFE TO WIN

KEEP ON PUSHING AND NEVER GIVE UP!

Ace McCloud

Be sure to check out my website for all my Books and Audio books.

www.AcesEbooks.com

Introduction

I want to thank you and congratulate you for buying the book, "Acid Reflux Cure: How To Treat Acid Reflux, How To Prevent Acid Reflux, All Natural Remedies For Acid Reflux, Medical Breakthroughs For Acid Reflux, And Proper Diet And Exercise For Acid Reflux."

This book contains proven steps and strategies on how to prevent, deal with, and cure Acid Reflux Disease. If you suffer from this condition, this book is a must read as you know just how distressing and painful it can be.

Don't burn another minute; start reading today and take charge of your destiny. Find out what triggers heartburn and other Acid Reflux Disease symptoms so you will know what foods, beverages and activities to avoid. Learn remedies, both medical and alternative, that will help you be proactive in the war that rages deep within. Suffer no more. There is help.

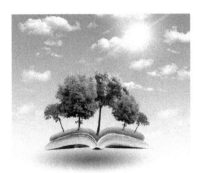

Chapter 1: Acid Reflux Disease: What Fuels the Fire?

Do you, or anyone you know, suffer from Acid Reflux Disease? If so, you know just how miserable it can be. According to the latest studies, the National Digestive Diseases Information Clearing house (NDDIC) has reported that at least 20 percent of Americans suffer from reflux symptoms at least once a week. Of those, every year 4.7 million require hospitalization and 1,653 die from the disease.

Acid Reflux Disease, or Gastroesophageal Reflux Disease (GERD), is a chronic condition that occurs when the lower esophageal sphincter allows gastric acids to enter up into the esophagus. Simply put, it is when stomach acids flow into the esophagus regularly.

An Australian physician named Dr. Barry Marshall discovered even more about the condition in the early 1980's. He learned through countless studies that an organism called helicobacter pylori is responsible for a chronic inflammation in the stomach lining and that often it is the root of Acid Reflux Disease.

The symptoms caused by Acid Reflux Disease range from heartburn, acid indigestion, chest pain, nausea, and regurgitation. Other characteristics sometimes experienced with the condition include pain or difficulty with swallowing, increased saliva, sore throat, and coughing.

Although the disease is often minimalized, it is very painful and can be quite serious. Some of the negative consequences can be damage to the esophageal lining, ulcers, narrowing of the esophagus, loss of appetite, breathing problems, inflamed or infected lungs, shrinking of air passages, and even cancer of the esophagus.

With 20 out of every 100 Americans suffering from the disorder, you can just imagine the economic impact it has on our society. Billions of dollars are spent on hospitalization, doctor's visits, and prescriptions each year not to mention the catastrophic loss of work and the large number of disability claims that are a direct result of the condition.

Equally as distressing are the negative effects Acid Reflux Disease can have on the individual's quality of life. If you suffer from it, you know the toll it can take physically, mentally and emotionally. Stress and depression are common among those with the illness and complicate the issue as both stress and depression feed the disease and the disease feeds stress and depression. It is an endless cycle.

Whether mild or severe, long term or short, the repercussions not only damage your quality of life but your style of life as well. What you eat, what you drink and where you go are basically governed by the disease. Symptoms such as belching and passing gas are often related to the condition and are downright embarrassing. No one wants to be humiliated in public so it is easy to withdraw from daily activities and eventually from life itself.

Chapter 2: How to Prevent Acid Reflux Disease

An ounce of prevention is worth a pound of cure. You've heard the old adage a million times but it certainly rings true where Acid Reflux Disease is concerned. It is definitely best to take measures to avoid the disease totally, but if that cannot be done, it is smart to take measures to at least nip it in the bud before it is full-blown and really causing you some discomfort.

Keeping in mind that Acid Reflux disease is a condition that is caused by a malfunctioning esophageal sphincter, it can still be affected by a variety of factors including those that are environmental, genetic, and physiological in nature. It can also be affected by lifestyle choices. There are things that can be done to prevent the condition and to help ensure optimal digestive health.

Diet

First and foremost, the role your diet plays in your digestive health cannot be stressed enough. What you put into your body directly determines what you get out of it. In other words, you cannot have poor eating habits and expect to be in good health.

In addition to eating healthy, there are certain foods that can irritate Acid Reflux Disease even though they are nutritious. It is best to avoid fruits and vegetables that are high in acid such as lemons, oranges, grapefruits, tomatoes, and onions. What you drink is important too. Citrus juices, tomato juice, coffee, and other caffeinated beverages have been proven to increase the risk of the condition.

Some foods are known to weaken the lower esophageal sphincter muscle which is a ring of smooth muscle fibers that separates the esophagus from the stomach and keeps the stomach's contents from back flowing. If the muscle is not working properly, undigested foods, acids, and enzymes can escape, which results in Acid Reflux symptoms. Garlic and other spicy foods can cause malfunctioning, as can chocolate, fried foods, and many dairy products.

Then there are foods that are very beneficial to good digestive health and should be incorporated into your diet for prevention. Fiber-rich foods such as fruits, vegetables and whole grains are excellent because fiber assists the body in eliminating food faster. When food is removed from the body, toxins are removed as well, and when food and toxins spend less time in the digestive track, there is less risk of issues developing.

How you eat can determine how your food will digest. Eating smaller meals more frequently is a smart idea because when the stomach is full, it distends past its normal shape and size and the lower esophageal sphincter tends to relax and not do its job. Digestion works best in an upright position. Since the esophageal muscle is also inclined to weaken when you are lying down and stomach acids tend to flow more freely when you are lying down, it is wise to try and not lie down after eating and try not to eat too soon before bedtime.

Water

Drinking water can help prevent Acid Reflux. Although it may sound like a generic quick fix, too simple to really work, it's a scientific fact that water neutralizes stomach acids and helps to maintain a healthy balance between acidity and alkalinity. Furthermore, without an adequate supply of water, all bodily muscles and organs will begin to shut down, including those associated with digestive health such as the stomach, esophagus and lower esophageal sphincter.

Which water you drink does matter. Tap water is the main source of drinking water in the United States and is provided by public water systems which service 90 percent of the supply. The water is often polluted by lead, agricultural run offs and corrosion that can leak through the pipes.

Even the chemical disinfectants added to the water to make it safe are not safe. Some of the disinfectants themselves have harmful reactions when they mix with water's natural materials and produce harmful byproducts such as trihalomethane, bromate and haloacetic acids. Be sure to drink filtered water from a purification system or through bottled water. When choosing bottled water it is a good idea to check the PH level to make sure it has a PH value of 7 or higher. I am a big fan of the ZeroWater filter system and have been using it for the last four years with great success. I have tried some of the other cheaper methods of filtering water, but can always still taste the chemicals and other residues. I think ZeroWater is a great value and relatively inexpensive. When my filters are running low, I like to re-stock with the ZeroWater eight pack filters, as this will save money over the long term, and I tend to drink a lot of water.

How much water you consume is important too. The Institute of Medicine recommends that men drink at least 3 liters a day and 2.2 liters for women. Most people do not drink enough water even though they may think that they do, so it is a good idea to measure your daily intake. One of the very first thinks I do every day after waking up is I drink a huge glass of water, and sometimes I drink two huge glasses.

Exercise

An active lifestyle is certainly a great preventative measure to take. When you exercise regularly, you stand less chance for developing gastrointestinal disorders. For one, obese individuals are at higher risk for getting Acid Reflux Disease, so keeping your weight down is helpful for sure. Secondly, exercise is beneficial to the strengthening of organs and muscles involved in the digestive process so it helps enable them to do their jobs more efficiently.

Exercise boosts the immune system and when the immune system is working well, there is less chance disease of any kind will develop. Regular exercise also improves mental health and helps to fight off stress and depression which can irritate the digestive process and cause problems.

Some exercises are thought to be better than others for preventing gastrointestinal issues. Those done with jiggling and shaking may trigger a reflux reaction, so riding on a stationary bike would be more conducive than running. Likewise, exercises done in a horizontal position may also promote digestive problems, so doing exercises upright would be best.

Stress

Perhaps easier said than done, avoiding stress is a must when it comes to promoting a healthy digestive system and preventing disease. Stress provokes Acid Reflux Disease. When you are stressed, your body is far more likely to succumb to an illness. Stress also heightens the disease's symptoms like heartburn, nausea and acid indigestion.

Stress is at epidemic levels in America with 43 percent of the adult population suffering from negative stress effects. The American Institute of stress reports that 22 percent of 1,226 U.S. residents suffer from extreme stress. It is estimated that 75 to 90 percent of all doctor's office calls are due to stress-rooted ailments. Stress is a killer and something you should keep an eye on. Exercise is a great way to relieve stress, so if you find yourself overwhelmed, be sure to get your work out in!

The good news is that there are measures you can take before stress hits you in the gut. A positive approach to life on life's terms is helpful for sure. Some things in life will always be stressful like financial hardships, bills and some work situations. Other stress sources can be eliminated. It is a good idea to identify the things in your life that cause stress and to know which situations you can change and which you cannot.

Relaxation therapy, Yoga and even seeing a counselor are all great ways to take hold of stress before it takes hold of you. Life can get busy and overwhelming but the more you take time to unwind and distress, the better off your health will be. If you really want to bring some true joy and happiness into your life to help relieve stress you are feeling, be sure to check out my book: Laughter Therapy.

Smoking

It is a proven fact that smoking tobacco is linked to Acid Reflux Disease. Studies show that not only does nicotine cause conditions favorable to contracting the illness but symptoms are complicated by it as well. While some who suffer from gastrointestinal issues claim doing so is therapeutic because it relieves stress, in reality that is far from the truth.

Smoking relaxes the lower esophageal sphincter which is a ring of muscles that regulate the passing of food into the stomach. It also prevents acid from back flowing into the esophagus. When it is relaxed, it does not work properly and esophagus damage occurs.

Smoking actually encourages acid production in the stomach. It also causes the intestines to transfer bile salts into the stomach which results in more potent acid. With stomach acid being more abundant and in such strength, the chance of it backing into the esophagus is greatly increased.

Other ways smoking can lead to gastrointestinal distress is that it damages the mucus membranes that line the esophagus. Those membranes aid in protecting the esophagus from being damaged by digestive acids. Smoking and nicotine also reduce the production of saliva and since saliva contains bicarbonate, an acid-neutralizing substance, that can certainly cause problems.

If you want to help ensure you do not get Acid Reflux Disease, it is best not to smoke. If you do smoke and would like to quit, there are a number of things you can do to make doing so as comfortable as possible. For serious help in quitting smoking, be sure to check out my book: Quit Smoking Now Quickly And Easily.

Sleep

It is important to get plenty of sleep to defend against gastrointestinal malfunctions. According to a recent poll conducted by the National Sleep Foundation, it was found that American adults who suffer from gastrointestinal disease also suffer from sleep disorders like sleep apnea and insomnia. Digestive distress no doubt causes one to not be able to sleep and lack of sleep leaves one susceptible to digestive disorders, so the two go hand in hand.

When you sleep, you heal. Your body is designed to rejuvenate, refresh and restore itself while sleeping and when adequate time is not given for it to do so, the door is opened for all sorts of problems and gastrointestinal issues are at the top of the list.

The occurrence of acid refluxing actually happens considerably less while you are sleeping. The problem, however, is getting to sleep. When you are sitting or standing, gravity helps to keep the contents of the stomach down and away from the junction of the stomach and esophagus, but when you lay down, it is more likely that the acidy contents will overflow into the esophagus and cause reflux. This then can cause pain and discomfort, making it hard, if not impossible, to fall asleep.

One helpful solution is to eat a smaller meal before bedtime. Eating earlier is a good idea too. It is suggested that you don't lie down for at least two hours after a meal. Furthermore, taking a walk after you eat will help to get your digestive juices flowing in the right direction.

Another great tip is to elevate your upper body when you lay down to go to sleep. Propping up with pillows or slipping some books or a wedge under the head of your mattress provides one inexpensive solution. You can also purchase a special bed that elevates at the head of the bed to help keep your stomach contents down.

Chapter 3: Medical Solutions: When Enough is Enough

When the symptoms of Acid Reflux Disease are frequent or severe, it is time to seek help. If you have tried preventative measures to no avail, it is an indicator that your problem may require a more intensive treatment. Not only can the condition be miserable, but there can be serious underlying conditions as well.

Over-the-Counter Medications

Over-the-counter prescriptions are often helpful. There are a myriad of medicines available without a prescription. It is wise to learn about the various types and also about any health risk warnings and possible interactions they may pose when taken with other drugs. Be sure to check with your physician before taking any.

Antacids

Antacids are perhaps the most popular of the over-the-counter medicines available. Rolaids, Tums, Maalox, Mylanta, and Alka-Seltzer are some of the most common brands. Antacids neutralize stomach acid, therefore providing quick relief, but the results are short lived because they only put a band aid on the real problem. Although they help to reduce the amount of acid in the stomach and coat the esophageal lining, they do nothing for the actual inflammation of the lining.

Antacids are taken by mouth and are available in liquid, dissolvable and chewable forms. Most contain an added active ingredient such as aluminum, calcium, magnesium or sodium bicarbonate. The added ingredient is designed to enhance the antacid's performance, but each can cause side effects as well.

The fact of the matter is that although antacids are a temporary fix, there are times that any relief is better than none at all. Moderation is important because overuse can result in diarrhea, constipation, headaches and other unwanted side effects. If your symptoms persist or if you are relying on antacids on a regular basis, it's time to see your doctor.

Oral Suspension Medications

Oral suspension medications actually coat the inside of the esophagus to provide relief from acid indigestion and heartburn. Like antacids, they are available in liquid, dissolvable and chewable forms. Pepto Bismol and Carafate are two of the most popular brands.

Some who suffer from symptoms of Acid Reflux Disease find that oral suspension medications work better for them than antacids do because they do actually bathe

the esophageal lining. Like antacids, the fix is temporary, and can bring on side effects as well.

Anti-Gas Medications

Pressure, gas and bloating are indications associated with Acid Reflux Disease. These symptoms can be painful and embarrassing as well. Anti-gas medications work fast to eliminate the immediate problem by breaking up gas bubbles, but they do not heal the root problem.

Maalox and Mylanta are examples of anti-gas formulas. They are taken orally such as in liquid, chewable or dissolving forms so they can begin to work immediately. Other active ingredients commonly added in the medications are aluminum, magnesium and simethicone, which have beneficial properties as well as possible negative implications as well. Please see your doctor if you require relief from symptoms on a frequent or regular basis or are taking any other medications.

H-2 Receptor Blockers

H-2 Receptor Blocker is an antagonist that decreases the volume of acid that the stomach produces. By definition, an antagonist counteracts the action of another and that is exactly what this medication does. Histamine is a substance the body produces to fight tissue damage and allergic reactions. When histamine reaches the H-2 receptors, it stimulates acid production, which is why a blocker is so effective in an overly acidic stomach.

Although many find excellent relief with the outcome of H-2 Receptor Blockers, they are slow acting and should be taken before the onset of gastric distress. Pepcid AC and Zantac are two leading brands of H-2 receptor blockers and were once only available through a prescription, but are now accessible without one. H-2 Receptor Blockers are, as a rule, are generally well tolerated but can certainly have unwanted side-effects such as dizziness, confusion, headaches and rashes. They can also have possible negative side effects with other medicines being taken.

Proton Pump Inhibitors

Proton pump inhibitors block acid production in the stomach and actually help heal esophageal damage. This type of medication is becoming more and more popular for fighting gastrointestinal distress because it is very effective. Once only available by prescription, proton pump inhibitors are now sold over-the-counter.

Derivatives of benzimidazole or benzimidazole, the inhibitors are very potent and are preferred by many over the H-2 receptor blockers because they work quicker and more efficiently. It is important to remember, however, these are best used in advance, as they may not be as effective after acid reflux symptoms are already present. Prilosec and Prevacid are popular brands readily available.

15

Seeing a Physician

In the United States alone, 20% of people with Acid Reflux Disease have symptoms in a given week and 7% have them every day. When symptoms are once a week and especially when they are on a daily basis, it warrants seeing a doctor and it is best done sooner than later. The condition can have serious implications and can worsen if not treated.

Diagnosis

There are a number of questions your physician may ask and several tests he/she may administer in order to rule on a positive or negative diagnosis.

Prescribed Medications

One of the most effective ways a physician may diagnose Acid Reflux Disease is by prescribing a medication. If the symptoms are relieved by taking the medication, chances are high that the patient has the disease. If symptoms persist or more severe ones are noted, it is an indicator that the underlying problem is a complication of the condition, is more advanced or is an entirely different issue.

Prescribed medications for acid reflux are much like the over-the-counter ones. Anti-acids, oral suspension, anti-gas, H-2 receptor blockers and proton pump inhibitors are all available in prescription strengths. The doctor is then able to adjust your dosage, if needed, and also to monitor progress or the lack there of.

Tests

Esophagogastroduodenoscopy

An Esophagogastroduodenoscopy (upper endoscopy) may be done by inserting a small camera that examines the esophagus lining, stomach and the upper part of the small intestine. The procedure is minimally invasive and can provide very valuable information as to the nature of the digestive illness. Although the procedure is minimally invasive, it can be quite uncomfortable when it is being performed. A biopsy may or may not be done based on the recommendation from your doctor.

Barium Swallow Radiograph

A Barium Swallow Radiograph is an x-ray that is administered after drinking a barium solution. It is designed to look for structural abnormalities, erosion in the esophagus, hiatal hernia, ulcers and many other structural abnormalities. Although not pleasant, it is extremely useful for diagnosing acid reflux and will show things that an Esophagogastroduodenoscopy and Barium Swallow Radiograph will not.

Esophageal Manometry

An Esophageal Manometry is a procedure done with a catheter that is positioned into the nose and guided into the stomach. The test detects motility (spastic movements) and peristalsis (contractions) of the esophagus. It is typically done when symptoms include complaints of swallowing and it will measure the esophagus strength and muscle coordination when swallowing occurs.

Esophageal pH Monitoring

One of the most common as well as most effective diagnosis tests used to detect Acid Reflux Disease is Esophageal pH Monitoring. The direct detection and measurement of acid in the esophagus is collected by a device inserted into the esophagus and left in place for 1-2 days. Depending on the outcome, the physician will then make a recommendation as to treatment if excess acid is found.

Surgery

When medical therapy has failed, surgery may be required. Although many do find relief after an operation for Acid Reflux Disease, it is important to know that the surgery does not necessarily alleviate all of the symptoms. Many patients still have to take prescribed medication for heartburn or acid control. The risks involved in gastric surgery are low but nonetheless, there are some and 10% of surgical patients have to undergo a repeat surgery.

Fundoplication

Fundoplication is the most common surgery for the disease. Of those surveyed who had the surgery after a five year period, 90% to 95% said they were pleased with the results and 80% reported feeling relief from their symptoms.

In this procedure, the lower esophageal sphincter is strengthened by wrapping the upper curve of the stomach around the esophagus and sewing it into place. With the esophageal sphincter able to function properly, it stops the backflow of acid. The operation can be an open surgery or laparoscopic. A laparoscopic surgery is less invasive and has a shorter recovery time.

Endoscopic Procedure

The Endoscopic Procedure allows the end of the esophagus to be bound to the top of the stomach without an incision. A small tube that contains a light, camera and small surgical tools is flexed through the mouth and on down into the esophagus and stomach. This is a minimally invasive operation that requires a short recovery time and has been found to be very effective.

Radiofrequency Treatment

Another treatment for Acid Reflux Disease is the Radiofrequency Treatment in which high-energy radio waves are sent into the lower esophagus wall. The waves cause the esophagus to produce small amounts of scar tissue which actually act as a barrier against the burning and irritation of the esophageal lining. Although the treatment is generally effective to a degree, it is not usually as successful as surgery and often has to be repeated. Still, it is desirable because it requires no incision, no hospital stay and little, if any, recuperation time.

Chapter 4: All Natural and Alternative Solutions

A growing number of the American population is turning to alternative methods of treating illnesses such as Acid Reflux Disease. A recent study shows that nearly 38% of adults and 12% of children have turned to Alternative Medicine.

Alternative Medicine, by definition, is products and practices used instead of traditional (standard) care such as family and specialized physicians, doctors of osteopathy and physical therapists. Homeopathy, chiropractic, herbal supplementation, meditation, osteopathic manipulation and acupuncture are examples of Alternative Treatments. When Traditional Medicine is used along with Alternative Treatments, it is referred to as Complementary Medicine.

Why do people use alternative options to conventional medicines and treatments? Of course the belief and hope is that a particular alternative method will work is the main reason, but equally as important is that many believe traditional treatment does not work or even worse, causes more harm than good. Many have had bad experiences with prescription drug side effects, dealt with bum surgeries or have simply had no good fortune with conventional methods.

There are four basic categories in Alternative Treatment. Biologically Based Practices supplement a healthy diet with particular foods, extracts, herbs or nutrients that are intended to heal or improve a condition. Manipulative therapy, also known as Manual Therapy or Body Based Therapy, concentrates on physical treatment where the body's structures and systems are manipulated, massaged or moved in some manner to promote healing. Techniques that are Mind-Body Therapies work to connect mind, spirit and body into harmony and whole health such as Biofeedback and Yoga. Energy therapies are designed to channel energy to restore health.

Biological Based Practices

Aloe Vera

As simple as it may sound, the Aloe Vera plant is praised by many who suffer from symptoms of Acid Reflux Disease. Just as the product soothes burned or irritated skin externally, it is used in drinkable form to heal acid burns in the digestive areas, restoring damaged tissue from the inside out. It is said to eliminate heartburn, gas, bloating, and even constipation and one reason is that it not only promotes healing of burns caused by stomach acid but it also helps at the root of the problem in actually balancing stomach acidity.

Throughout history, the Aloe Vera plant has been used for medicinal purposes with written records dating back as far as 512 AD. It is not only available in its natural state but in liquid and pill form as well. Although the plant's healing properties have been proven, it can be lethal in high doses and should be taken with caution. Aloe Vera juice is my favorite method for combatting my acid reflux. Fruit of the Earth makes a great and very inexpensive Aloe Vera juice that you can get at Walmart or at Walmart online. It is under eight dollars a gallon, which is a great price. Fruit of the Earth Aloe Vera Juice. It is recommended that you take ½ cup of the juice before each meal, and you can take shot glass sized doses whenever you feel that you may need it. I think Aloe Vera juice should be the first thing you get for a super healthy and all natural solution. Ever since I started drinking Aloe Vera Juice regularly I have had almost no problems with acid reflux.

Honey

Honey can be great for relieving acid reflux symptoms. Just take one teaspoon of raw, pure honey whenever you feel that you may need it or when discomfort occurs. Right before bedtime is another great time to take a dose of honey as well. Ambrosia honey company makes a great product. Taking honey regularly along with Aloe Vera juice can be extremely beneficial to helping with acid reflux.

Licorice

Licorice is a popular natural supplement for digestive disorders. The main ingredient of licorice root, Glycyrrhiza glabra, is known for its soothing properties and is said to help intestines, stomach, throat and lungs, all which can be affected by Acid Reflux Disease. Licorice also inhibits Helicobacter pylori which is a micro bacteria found in the stomach lining of a large majority of people who suffer from gastrointestinal problems.

Apples

Apples can bring great relief from acid reflux symptoms. Red delicious, golden delicious, and Braeburn apples are the best. Eat an apple when you're feeling discomfort and right before bedtime is a good time to eat them as well.

Vinegar

You can take 1 to 2 tablespoons of vinegar with your meals to help reduce any flare-ups that you may have.

Slippery Elm

Slippery elm, Ulmus rubra, is a natural supplement that has many uses as an herbal remedy including digestive disorders. The main component of slippery elm is mucilage which is a demulcent, a substance that sooths and heals by forming a film over a mucous membrane. It also decreases inflammation.

Since Acid Reflux Disease symptoms often include irritation, inflammation and burning of the esophageal lining and other membranes, slippery elm is can be very beneficial for those problems and it also encourages the nerve endings to reflux, which in turn causes them to produce more mucus ,which acts to prevent an overabundance of acid. Tablets, capsules, powder, lozenges, and teas are the most common ways slippery elm is taken and relief is generally felt almost immediately.

Red Grape juice and Pectin

Put ½ teaspoon of pectin in a glass of red grape juice and drink when symptoms flare up.

Zinc and L-Carnosine

These two supplements, when taken together, help to protect the lining of the stomach. You can also purchase them already mixed together in a product called: Nature's Lining. This is a good product to try if you have a more severe case of acid reflux.

Peppermint

One of the most popular, yet controversial, herbal remedies is peppermint which is a plant well known for its medicinal uses. The leaves can be chewed or made into tea or oil. Capsules and pills are also available but lozenges are the favorite form of ingestion due to its desirable taste. Although peppermint is used for gastrointestinal issues, it is not tolerated well by some sufferers and should be taken with caution.

Baking Soda and Water

Add 1 teaspoon of baking soda to a glass of water and drink when symptoms flare up.

Green Tea with Ginseng

Drinking green tea with ginseng has been shown to give relief to some people.

Manipulative Therapy

Massage

Tension of the stomach and diaphragm can be released by gentle osteopathic movement and massage. Tension of the digestive areas affected by Acid Reflux Disease can also cause unaffected areas to become tense, such as the spine and neck, so movement and massage on those places can be helpful as well. Therapeutic oils can be used to help to relax and revive the gastrointestinal organs and tissues. If you would like to know how to massage yourself or others be sure to check out my book: The Best of Massage, Trigger Point, and Acupressure Therapy.

Chiropractic Procedures

In addition to spine and neck issues, Chiropractic Procedures have been credited to helping with digestive problems as well. Although it may seem odd, the nerves in the mid-back area work directly with your upper digestive track and stomach. When the nerves become irritated, inflamed or compacted, the nerves can cease to function correctly causing a number of gastrointestinal problems.

Restoring spinal health and alignment does a number of things to help with Acid Reflux symptoms. It can aid in stomach functions but also can correct hiatal hernias which happen when the top of the stomach pushes through the valve releasing acid into the stomach. In addition, there are nerves in the base of the neck and between the shoulder blades that work with the muscles used to swallow. The nerves often become damaged and strained, but through Chiropractic manipulation, these nerves can be corrected.

It is important to note that Chiropractic help will most likely not happen in just one adjustment. Often it takes up to three months or longer to fully experience the benefits. Combining Chiropractic therapy with good nutrition, supplements and positive health habits will produce optimal results.

Energy Therapy

Magnet Therapy

The use of static magnetic fields as a treatment is called Magnet Therapy, or Magnotherapy. Practitioners believe that disruption of energy in the body's cells results in a faulty metabolism which can mean the cells are not healthy. Since energy is electromagnetic in nature, the concept is that by applying magnetic fields to the body, it will help those targeted areas receive healing benefits. In addition to the re-energizing of cells, blood flow is increased to the impaired tissues through magnetic energy.

There are various methods that Magnetic Therapy can be used for Acid Reflux Disease in particular. The treatment is often used to increase the production of acid in the stomach during mealtime so that the gastric acid actually helps digest the food as it is intended to do. Another focus is to speed the digestion process thus decreasing the time reflux could occur. In addition to the stomach, the magnetic field can be placed over the lower esophagus or the upper abdomen once digestion has taken place with the goal of eliminating or at least relieving heartburn and other symptoms of the condition.

Many Magnotherapy products are on the market today. Bracelets and other jewelry, blankets, mattresses and even creams are made with claims that they have therapeutic levels of magnetic energy in them. There are also bands available that can be worn on various parts of the body such as wrists, fingers, feet and even stomachs.

Numerous studies have been conducted on the subject of magnetic therapy but none are conclusive one way or the other except for the LINX Reflux

Management System which is a magnetic device implanted in the lower esophageal sphincter through a laparoscopic surgery. The LINX system consists of titanium beads with magnetic cores that are placed in a ring and are connected with wires of titanium.

The FDA approved treatment is reported to have a 64% success rate with patients either feeling completely normal or at least considerably improved. The procedure generally takes less than an hour, has a very short recovery time and is minimally invasive.

Acupuncture

Acupuncture is a form of Energy Therapy that uses needles that are placed in the skin with the intention of opening channels that are blocked in order to restore health. An ancient Chinese practice, Acupuncture is becoming increasingly popular for ailments such as Acid Reflux Disease.

Studies have shown that certain points on the wrist are in direct relation to the esophageal sphincter, the muscle band responsible for preventing stomach acids from back flowing into the esophagus. When these points are re-energized, it is said that the body can be restored to health. Acupuncture is also known to relax the body and relive stress so that digestive disorders brought on or worsened by tension can be made better.

As with Chiropractic Treatment, Acupuncture Therapy cannot be expected to show results overnight. It often takes multiple sessions. A healthy lifestyle certainly enhances the benefits of Acupuncture and will help the chances that the treatment will work.

Mind-Body Therapy

Yoga

Yoga is a discipline that deals with mind, soul and body. It is an ancient practice that dates back to as late as 500-200 BC. The therapy routine is designed to not only spiritually enhance a person's wellbeing, but to physically strengthen and tone muscles and to relieve tension and stress.

Yoga is very good for the spine and since all functions of the body stem from the spine, most yoga exercises will benefit the digestive areas. There are even postures that focus specifically on helping acid indigestion and heartburn. Many have found the practice of Yoga relieves or eliminates symptoms of Acid Reflux Disease and brings about whole body health at the same time. Here is a great video on YouTube by Yoga with Adriene, Yoga for Acid Reflux – Embrace It!, telling how to do some yoga exercises for acid reflux.

Biofeedback

Biofeedback is a system used to gather and use information which is physiological roots of a physical or emotional condition. Generally, but not always, special equipment is used to perform the therapy. Once the knowledge is attained, it can be used to control the problematic areas by use of brainwaves, heart rate and muscle tone. Basically, it is retraining the body to act and react in a better and healthier manner. This type of treatment is especially useful for conditions that stem from stress and anxiety or psychological issues.

Since Acid Reflux Disease is caused or complicated by emotional, mental and physical strain, Biofeedback can be very helpful for manipulating thoughts, emotions and behaviors in order to bring a person to a better state of being. With successful treatment, symptoms that originate or are aggravated by stress can hopefully be alleviated.

Chapter 5: Exercise: The Skinny on the Burn

When it comes to Acid Reflux Disease, exercise can be a positive or a negative, the cause or the cure. Regular exercise can help prevent gastrointestinal issues and even treat symptoms when they occur. On the other hand, exercise induced or exercise aggravated reflux is equally as common.

ON A POSITIVE NOTE

The right exercises done at the right time can be very conducive for Acid Reflux Disease issues. Studies have proven that moderate exercise done a few times a week cut can actually greatly reduce the chance of getting the condition. For those who already suffer, regular exercise greatly helped with the symptoms.

WEIGHT

Being obese increases one's chances for experiencing Acid Reflux Disease. In fact, those who are extremely overweight triple their chance of having the condition. Of those who do suffer, their symptoms are oftentimes greater and more severe.

HEALTH

Exercise is instrumental in maintaining a proper weight which, in turn, helps the muscular valve at the end of the gullet, the esophageal sphincter, to remain shut so digestive acids do not back flow. In addition, exercise makes for healthy functions of muscles and organs so the benefits are many when it comes to the entire digestion system.

DIET

It is important to pay attention to your diet. Waiting at least two hours after a meal to exercise is advised or to exercise on an empty stomach altogether. If you do choose to eat, a banana or yogurt is a wise choice. High carbohydrate sports drinks can aggravate acid conditions so those are best avoided. Spicy or high acidic foods or beverages should be eliminated as well.

WISE EXERCISE

Vigorous exercises, like running and jumping, can create heartburn in healthy individuals so it can certainly impair those with gastrointestinal issues. Substitute strenuous exercises for those that are more stationary such as cycling. Routines that involve lying flat on your back are more likely to cause problems. Leg curls and bench presses are not conducive while Yoga type exercises are wonderful options.

As mentioned above, too much moving, jumping and running can not only burn calories but burn your intestinal organs as well. Acid Reflux Disease can be complicated and provoked by exercises that bounce the digestive acids around and this type of exercise can also bring on acid reflux symptoms for those who generally do not experience them. It is important to realize, though, how vital exercise is to the prevention and possible cure of acid reflux, so focus on finding exercise that work for you.

Chapter 6: Dietary Solutions

What to eat and what not to eat, that is the dilemma. Diet is perhaps the most important thing to take into consideration when dealing with GERD. Like exercise, it can provoke or prevent and symptoms. It is imperative to research the facts so you can help yourself rather than hurt yourself by what you eat and drink.

What to Eat

Choosing healthy foods that do not cause Acid Reflux Disease symptoms just makes common sense. Low-fat, high-protein meals are optimal especially when eaten in smaller more frequent meals.

Bananas

Bananas are great for gastrointestinal issues because they have a pH 5.6, making them easily digestible for most people. A select few of those who suffer with Acid Reflux Disease, however, cannot tolerate bananas.

Oatmeal

Oatmeal is a fantastic and nutritious food that does not promote acid indigestion. It is chalk full of vitamins and also contains a water soluble fiber that helps to slow digestion. Oatmeal, cooked or uncooked, has low acidity and digests easily.

Ginger

Ginger not only does not agitate digestive disorders, it actually treats the symptoms. A natural anti-inflammatory, ginger has been used medicinally for hundreds of years. Ginger comes in crystalized or powder form but also as a root that can be grated, diced, peeled and sliced. It can be pickled, steeped or simply used as an ingredient in a dish. You can also take it in capsule form. Here is a great choice if you would like to add a ginger supplement to your diet: Nature's Way Ginger Supplement.

WHAT TO AVOID

Caffeine and Carbonation

It may also help to avoid certain beverages and foods that trigger heartburn symptoms and those that make the symptoms worse. Both coffee and tea, caffeinated and decaffeinated, are known to cause acid reflux. Most caffeinated and carbonated beverages aggravate the condition and should be avoided as well. Ginger-ale is perhaps one exception to the rule.

Alcohol

A recent study showed that heavy drinkers were three times more likely to have acid reflux than individuals who do not drink alcohol. One reason for this is that alcohol can inflame the internal organs and also can relax the muscle that holds the acid intact.

Citrus Fruits and Juices

Citrus foods are high in acid and can certainly bring on indigestion complications so it is best to avoid these fruits and juices. In addition, acid relaxes the lower esophageal sphincter so stomach juices can more easily backwash and cause issues.

Tomatoes and Tomato Sauces

Tomatoes and tomato sauces are high in acid and can cause indigestion and relax the esophageal sphincter just like citrus foods so these should be avoided or consumed in moderation.

Chocolate

Chocolate, both milk and dark, does not set well with those who have digestion problems and the main reason why is that chocolate contains theobromine, a compound that triggers the esophageal sphincter muscles to relax. When that happens, stomach acids escape and cause heartburn.

Mint and Peppermint

Contrary to popular belief, mints are not good for acid reflux and in fact, mints are an irritant to the condition. Although they may soothe initially, mints of any kind do more harm than good and should be avoided.

Spicy and Fatty Foods

Spicy foods are irritating to those suffering from Acid Reflux Disease as are foods that are high in fat. Avoid chili peppers, curry and the likes as well as fatty meats and high fat dairy.

Onion and Garlic

Onion and garlic set fire to the digestion process and usually do so almost immediately after being eaten. If you are set on having them, try sautéing them before consuming to lessen the burn, but they are best left out the diet of a person who suffers from acid reflux.

Chapter 7: Water: Tap In or Tap Out

Drink Up!

It only makes sense that water is one of the best cures for Acid Reflux Disease. As mentioned early in the book, drinking water is a great prevention, but it is a cure as well.

Studies actually show that water increases gastric pH more effectively than acid inhibiting drugs. It works faster too. While drugs such as antacid, ranitidine, omeprazole, rabeprazole and esomeprazole took over 4 minutes, water took less than 1. Water is a lot cheaper and has no side effects.

Our body needs water to function properly. The more water you drink, the better your bodily organs and muscles work and the better you will be able to digest. When you do not consume enough water, your body goes into dehydration mode which causes kinks in the system, especially in your digestive areas. Drinking plenty of water helps your body function like a well-oiled machine.

Water is the best option. When faced with the dilemma of what to drink, water wins. Carbonated and caffeinated beverages irritate digestive issues as do many juices and sometimes even milk, so play it safe and drink a big glass of water.

Is All Water Created Equally?

Tapping In

No. Water is not created the same. Practically all water that comes from the tap is toxic. It is not safe. There are chemicals, detergents, chlorine, and many other pollutants that are proven to be in the public water systems, so steer clear and do not drink tap water unless it is filtered.

Bottled Water

Bottled water is a good option, but again, not all bottled water is created equally. Some bottled waters contain fluoride, chlorine, and other ingredients not mentioned on the label. There are only a handful of bottled waters that actually list the ingredients and source of their water and are totally transparent about their product so these are the best ones to choose.

Filtration Systems

Having a home filtration system is the best way to assure that your water is safe for drinking. Carbon filtration and reverse osmosis are examples of filtering mechanisms that rid the water of pollutants and heavy metals. Be sure to do your homework if you opt to purchase one and then have the water tested once you put it in to be certain that it works. A simpler solution is to just use the ZeroWater pitcher. I have tried almost every water system there is out there and am quite pleased with the ZeroWater system and have been using it for the last three years.

29

When In Hot Water

It is not unusual for Acid Reflux Disease sufferers to complain that water actually worsens their symptoms. That creates a huge problem. Our bodies must have water to function and those who have problems such as digestive issues, may even need more water than most. What to do?

If your acid reflux is aggravated by water, try sipping it instead of guzzling. It may also help to drink water on a full, rather than an empty stomach and believe it or not, the more you drink, the more your body will be able to handle it. Sometimes the distress you may feel is your body coming out of dehydration mode. Do whatever works for you but do be sure to drink plenty of water.

Conclusion

I hope this book was able to help you to overcome your Acid Reflux Disease and to enjoy your life without the misery you once suffered from. Whether you choose to take the reins by seeing a physician, going the alternative route or any of the other solutions mentioned in this book, I am confident you will now make an informed decision and tackle the problem head on.

The next step is to maintain your health and take the steps necessary to live a healthy lifestyle that is conducive to remaining free from acid reflux. It's up to you. You can do it!

Finally, if you discovered at least one thing that has helped you or that you think would be beneficial to someone else, be sure to take a few seconds to easily post a quick positive review. As an author, your positive feedback is desperately needed. Your highly valuable five star reviews are like a river of golden joy flowing through a sunny forest of mighty trees and beautiful flowers! *To do your good deed in making the world a better place by helping others with your valuable insight, just leave a nice review.*

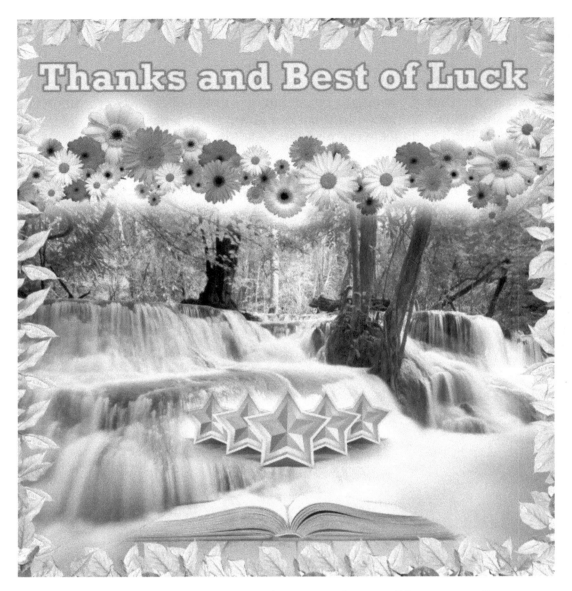

My Other Books and Audio Books
www.AcesEbooks.com

Health Books

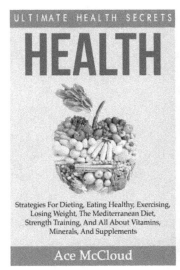

ULTIMATE HEALTH SECRETS

HEALTH

Strategies For Dieting, Eating Healthy, Exercising, Losing Weight, The Mediterranean Diet, Strength Training, And All About Vitamins, Minerals, And Supplements

Ace McCloud

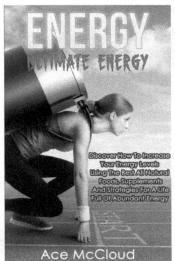

ENERGY
ULTIMATE ENERGY

Discover How To Increase Your Energy Levels Using The Best All Natural Foods, Supplements And Strategies For A Life Full Of Abundant Energy

Ace McCloud

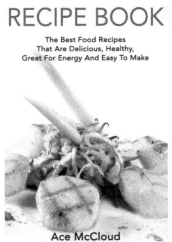

RECIPE BOOK

The Best Food Recipes That Are Delicious, Healthy, Great For Energy And Easy To Make

Ace McCloud

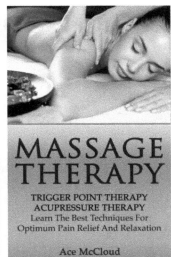

MASSAGE THERAPY

TRIGGER POINT THERAPY
ACUPRESSURE THERAPY
Learn The Best Techniques For Optimum Pain Relief And Relaxation

Ace McCloud

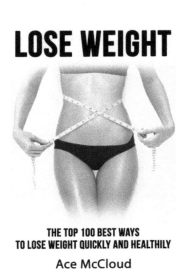

LOSE WEIGHT

THE TOP 100 BEST WAYS
TO LOSE WEIGHT QUICKLY AND HEALTHILY

Ace McCloud

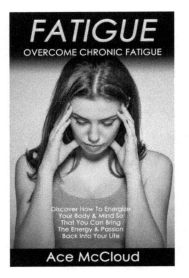

FATIGUE
OVERCOME CHRONIC FATIGUE

Discover How To Energize
Your Body & Mind So
That You Can Bring
The Energy & Passion
Back Into Your Life

Ace McCloud

Peak Performance Books

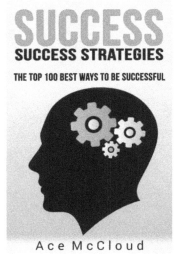

SUCCESS
SUCCESS STRATEGIES

THE TOP 100 BEST WAYS TO BE SUCCESSFUL

Ace McCloud

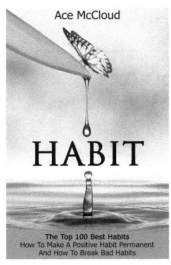

Ace McCloud

HABIT

The Top 100 Best Habits
How To Make A Positive Habit Permanent
And How To Break Bad Habits

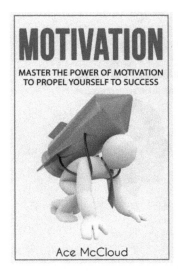

MOTIVATION

MASTER THE POWER OF MOTIVATION
TO PROPEL YOURSELF TO SUCCESS

Ace McCloud

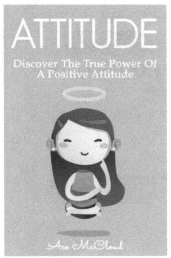

ATTITUDE

Discover The True Power Of
A Positive Attitude

Ace McCloud

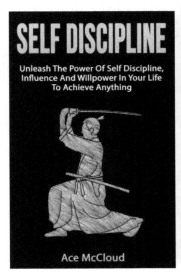

SELF DISCIPLINE

Unleash The Power Of Self Discipline,
Influence And Willpower In Your Life
To Achieve Anything

Ace McCloud

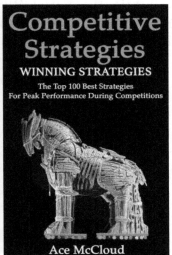

Competitive Strategies

WINNING STRATEGIES

The Top 100 Best Strategies
For Peak Performance During Competitions

Ace McCloud

Be sure to check out my audio books as well!

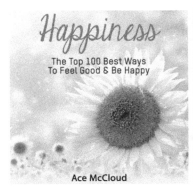

Happiness

The Top 100 Best Ways
To Feel Good & Be Happy

Ace McCloud

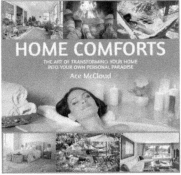

HOME COMFORTS

THE ART OF TRANSFORMING YOUR HOME
INTO YOUR OWN PERSONAL PARADISE

Ace McCloud

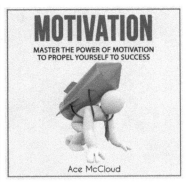

MOTIVATION

MASTER THE POWER OF MOTIVATION
TO PROPEL YOURSELF TO SUCCESS

Ace McCloud

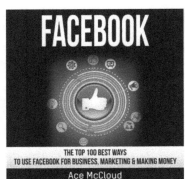 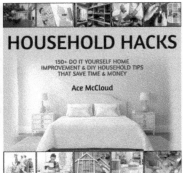 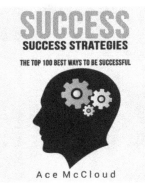

Be sure to check out my website at: **www.AcesEbooks.com** for a complete list of all of my books and high quality audio books. I enjoy bringing you the best knowledge in the world and wish you the best in using this information to make your journey through life better and more enjoyable! **Best of luck to you!**

CPSIA information can be obtained
at www.ICGtesting.com
Printed in the USA
BVHW012334140922
647051BV00004BA/106

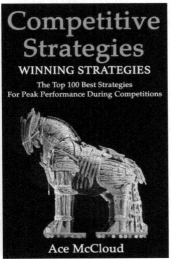